Offshore Race Food

Eating Well in Challenging Sailboat Conditions

Stephanie York

ISBN:
ISBN-978-0-9896252-1-0

DEDICATION

I dedicate this book to my daughter Amada York who pushes me to challenge myself and my husband Mark Coleman who supports me in my sometimes silly decisions. Thank you both and I love you!

CONTENTS

ACKNOWLEDGMENTS

I would like to acknowledge everyone who I have raced and sailed with, George Finch for being so patient on the bow, Jane Thomas who is the fearless captain of an amazing crew of women sailors where I learned to love sailing and the ladies of Sistership, Michelle Boronski, Johanna Gabbard who gave me the chance to be a part of the amazing R2AK race and Stephanie "We will always have the Rucus" Mahue who was a lot of fun.

Photo Credit

BACK COVER PHOTO BY BRONNY DANIELS
WWW.JOYSAILING.COM

Foreword

Originally this book was written for my husband and the team on the Trans Pac Race in 2011. I have left that section in its entirety for anyone who is making whole meals for a race boat with plenty of room on it, one fridge and a freezer with a secondary cooler/freezer as back up. It is the second half of this book. Since then I have pursued a racing career of my own and now have an additional section on providing food for the Race to Alaska on a trimaran named Sistership.com. You can look the race up at r2ak.com and on the Facebook page Race to Alaska by Northwest Maritime Center. It is an amazing race and a ton of fun to follow June of each year. Become a tracker junkie if you want, many people get addicted to following the boats. Pick a favorite and jump on board!

The addition in the beginning of the book is about dehydrating for the Race to Alaska. Limited space and the fact we were rowing the boat whenever we weren't sailing meant we had to keep weight down and conserve compartment use. So dehydrated food was the best choice on this race for us. I did a ton of research and the following is what I came up with that helped us. Enjoy!

This section includes chapters on prepping for the race, researching recipes, equipment, time required to rehydrate as well as the recipes I used. Enjoy and feel free to contact me anytime at slyohio@hotmail.com with questions you may have.

⛵ Chapter 1

About the R2AK Race and Food

It's been a little while since we finished the race, June 2017. Since then in 2018 an all-women's crew on Team Sail Like A Girl won the race in a mono-hull! So exciting. Love to see women doing well in sailboat racing, keep going for it!

On Team Sistership.com, aging proud and growing bold, we raced the R2AK in 2017. We came in 15th and are darn proud we finished at all. It was a tough year and we had mishaps for sure. We started with a crew of 4 on an F-27 Corsair Trimaran and finished with a crew of 3 in 12 ½ days, gale force events notwithstanding. The physical prep and journey is probably best left to another book. It was high winds, high seas, tons of rowing and a lot of great memories.

I do know that provisioning for the boat was a bit tougher than the Trans Pacific Race. We needed to keep weight down and spirits up as well as having enough nutrition to get through the grueling schedule. I knew what I needed to eat, high protein and no wheat, so I just made the type of food I needed and wanted, making enough for everyone. Following should be a description of how I figured out what we needed, where we would put it and how I got it done.

The Race, a crazy challenge

If you haven't heard of the R2AK race before you should go over and check out their website. It is an exciting site to see and will ratchet up the enthusiasm of anyone who likes to sail and race. The website is www.R2AK.com and their Facebook page is Race to Alaska by Northwest Maritime Center. Many of the teams have their own Facebook pages also and there are several documentaries and short clips about it on the web. Well worth looking at all the years, teams and posts.

As they explain it: "It's like the Iditarod, on a boat, with a chance of drowning, being run down by a freighter, or eaten by a grizzly bear. There are squalls, killer whales, tidal currents that run 20 miles an hour, and some of the most beautiful scenery in the world."
www.r2ak.com/about/r2ak-explained/

There are as many boats as there are sailors, every kind of experience level and a lot of excited fans. With the race ahead of us we had to figure out how to provision. In 2016 the same boat with 4 women did the race but they ate mostly dehydrated foods that were donated. These were the types of meals back packers take with them on long hikes. Because they were manufactured they had no control over the contents. Though the food was not bad it was bad for them.

The lack of variety caused them to not eat enough calories. The sodium content in the food caused severe swelling by the end of their 12th day and the cost of having to buy these ourselves with no donations was pretty steep for what appeared to be unhealthy outcomes. I knew I needed to make wholesome healthy food or I for one would not be of much use later on in the race.

So, I had provisioned for a long open ocean race before, the Trans Pac, as is covered in the second part of this book. I heard some friends of the team were making us some food as their donation to the team but it was made from pre-dehydrated mixes that were then added together. For my own nutrition I needed to have a blend of more complex foods and nutrients. I am not a picky eater, or maybe I am and don't know it, but I need to have high protein, low sugar and I have a wheat allergy. I let the team know I was going to be making my own food and they asked that I make more for everyone. Below is how I did it for our boat and some suggestions for your boat if you need any.

⛵Chapter 2

The Team – Owner and 3 crew

The team consisted of the captain, 1st mate, one crew and myself.

There were four of us to start and we lost a crew member about 100 miles into the race. Starting off I had planned meals to supplement the ones given to us by friends. Out of the team of four I was the only one that had food restrictions or needs. I eat wheat free due to a wheat sensitivity and I need high protein for the amount of physical activity we were going to be going through. No one else said they wanted anything in particular. We were planning for 14 days of racing, so enough food for us to eat that many days is actually a lot.

Here are some things to think about for the crew and planning:

1. Food Restrictions-allergies

Ask your team and the crew what food restrictions they have if any. Do they want to have nut free food, no gluten, low sugar.

2. Also ask what kinds of foods the individuals would like to eat.

Pick up on any of their likes, cravings and different things that will motivate them to eat enough, flavors such as Indian, Asian, spicy, sweet etc..

Keep in mind this is a very physically exerting race. What will the team need to keep going in extreme conditions? Will you need to have higher protein in all of the food? Do you need to limit sweets in food and have them as a snack only. I personally am weaker from sweets and have to focus on more complex carbohydrates so the food was critical. Everyone is a little different.

It really helps to have a variety of dishes to make it interesting at 3 AM when its freezing outside and you can't see the shore with logs floating all around. Things that are hot and tasty will get you through a midnight rowing session better than something you have already eaten 50 times. If one team member wants spicy but another doesn't consider spice packets or hot sauce.

3. How many crew will there be and how many days are you planning to sail? This will help with calculations on how much food to prep. Make a little extra, this has helped both times I prepped for a race.

⛵Chapter 3

The Boat, Galley and Equipment

The boat was an F-27 Corsair Trimaran. It had a lot more room than many of the boats who were sailing in the race. Seriously, you have got to go to the website and see all of these boats! Some only had a tarp for protection or in the case of the standup paddle boarder nothing. We had two berths down below with lee cloths and a little sink with a single burner that was strapped on top. We didn't know what the conditions would be but since the boat and captain had done the race the year before they knew what worked.

Figure out where on the boat you can have a burner, somewhere to heat water, store the water. Can you strap it down? Can you heat water while you are at anchor or underway, what would this look like? Practice using the cooking equipment during your practice sails. Nothing can replace real life practice. Heated water can be put into a tight container for later use once you are under way again.

Things to do before the race:

1. Measure all the space you can find to store food and equipment. Make sure you talk to the captain and crew to clear the use of this space for food so it is not going to being used for anything else.

    a. On the F27 we had cubby holes under the seats that worked perfect for storing bags of food. They would be stored at the water line and stay cool as well as be corralled and out of the way.

    b. Look on the walls as well. Can you lash a bag of provisions to the wall with Velcro or tie it up out of the way? Dehydrated bags can be squished really flat.

    c. Make sure you can secure the food firmly. The last thing you need is to have a bag of loose food crashing around when you hit a wall of wind or big waves.

    d. Keep track of everywhere the food has been stashed. Make one person in charge of knowing where it is all at. Some boats have a lot less room than others so you may have to be super creative which means you might forget where the chocolate bars are. Not good!

2. Find packaging that will work for those spaces, can you fit in a small box somewhere? We used a large plastic bag to hold the different smaller vacuum sealed bags inside. We separated the smaller bags into big bags based on lunch, breakfast and flavor profiles.

The Equipment

On our boat we heated up water on a burner using a 1 burner stove that held a propane can inside, they cost from 20 to 40 dollars. We used a tea kettle that would whistle when it was hot. After the water was hot we would then pour it into a large carafe with the push-top pour mechanism that was strapped onto our step up out of the galley so it would stay hot and available in all types of weather but not roll around when we hit the next gale force winds.

If you have a mono-hull the heel will be much more significant than the trimaran, practice in high wind with your equipment if you can. That way everything we ate or drank used the hot water. We took turns making more water. We had storage at the sink area where we could stow the food containers and utensils.

Again, this was a luxury, many of the competitors did not have a down below at all, no berth, no stove, no nothing, Crazies! (but they were awesome all the same!)

We used Screw top containers, specifically Makexpress 16oz double walled wide mouth sealable containers from Amazon, that could hold enough liquid to rehydrate each portion of food pre-sealed in their packets. You could fill it with water and let it sit anywhere without spilling so it could rehydrate and be ready to eat in 20-30 minutes.

It was as easy as cutting the sealed meal packets, dumping them into the containers, adding water to the top and waiting 20 minutes. The double wall made it easy to keep the food warm if you couldn't get to it too fast and the wide mouth opening helped a lot with eating the food and rinsing them out quickly with sea water, we could conserve fresh water that way.

Our water bottles also had carabiners on them so when we took them top side they could stay attached to the net or lines on the boat. Each team member had separate sporks with our name written on them as well as our own hot mug, water bottle and a sealable container with our names on stickers on each of them or written in permanent ink.

Look in the boat for small cubby holes, anywhere will work to stash food, snacks choose what will fit and then pick what you will want to take with you, we had tea, coffee, hot chocolate (big ticket item that one) as well as snacks of all kinds, crunchy salty and sweet are good for staying awake. We put them in containers and zip lock bags with writing on the side so we could grab them when we needed them under way. You could even put the bags of food or snacks into dry bags and toss them up into the sail area. Keeping your excess out of the way helps a lot when you are under way.

Notes:

⛵Chapter 4

The Budget

This is a big concern for all sailors when planning for a race. I did not keep track of all of my expenses so I cannot give a dollar amount for the food we took.

However, the year before they had back packing food pouches donated and if they had to buy them it would have been anywhere from 5 to 9 dollars per pouch per person per meal. This type of food also has a lot of sodium in it. The team had major edema from the salt in the food the year before so I knew this was not a good option for us.

I shopped for discounts and on sale items when I made my meals so I am sure the costs were significantly lower than they would have been if I bought from a company. We planned for around $150 each for costs per crew member covering 14 days of food for the R2AK. I believe that you can keep it to that dollar amount for a crew of 4 if you are doing the cooking yourself and can borrow equipment.

Plan out your menu, look through grocery flyers and source as close as you can everything you will need to make the meals and package them. I am a big fan of spreadsheets. Use the recipes here for an example. If you need 2 pounds of ground beef what would that cost? Then cans of tomato sauce etc. You could have this all on a simple excel spreadsheet and figure out the ultimate cost then divide by team members.

I would also figure out what snacks you want ahead of time, they add up quickly and just shopping on a whim will make you buy more than you planned on.

Donations: I found it helps to be very specific about what you need and if someone wants to donate then they can get you a bag of small candy bars for example. The Hershey variety bag is a good one. This way you are letting them participate but you are also getting things you want and will use.

Budget notes:

1. Make a list of recipes

2. Create a spreadsheet to track what is needed for each recipe and costs

3. Add costs of dehydrator

4. Add costs of packaging equipment, the small seal bags cost a little bit.

5. Make a list of items needed based on recipes and pass these out to family, friends and volunteers who want to help purchase things for the team

6. Consider a surprise bag of fancy treats, this is in case the team is going through a tough time and can really help morale.

Notes:

Chapter 5

The Food

As much as I try to save money I needed to experiment with the dehydrator. I had never used one before so I purchased one. I did a lot of research and the amount of food I was going to make meant I needed to go with a larger dehydrator.

Things to look at when dehydrating food for the trip:

1. Research the type of food and equipment you will be needing.

2. Dehydrating machine – borrow one or buy one.

3. Spreadsheet for the cost of each meal.

4. Communicate with the team costs and how it will be broken down.

5. Set up a timeline for getting all of the food done, this can be way ahead of time also.

6. Enlist friends and volunteers to help you out.

7. Look up tasty menu ideas online and ask friends and family for their favorite recipes. Keep in mind ground meats work best, whole chunks of meat will not rehydrate well.

Take the time to watch a lot of reviews, see the videos posted by users for the different machines and choose one that will work for you. After watching a lot of videos I decided I really liked the Excalibur 9 tray dehydrator. This was roughly $250.00 plus $4 dollars for the non-stick sheets. There are cheaper and smaller dehydrators that sell for $60.00 so if you have more time until your event you can get a smaller one and do smaller batches. Maybe even borrow one first before buying.

I also used a vacuum sealing machine that the owner of the boat had. Borrow one of these too, they are perfect for space saving and food protection. Ask around, someone has it stored in their garage somewhere.

If you cannot get a vacuum sealer then you could also use plastic zip top bags, not as sturdy or space conscious though. I didn't want any air to be in with the food so the vacuum seal bags were great.

The dehydrator had 9 trays and I purchased 9 non-stick dehydrator sheets as well because I knew I was going to be dehydrating liquids. Then I needed to make the sheets hold the liquid so I used binder clips from my office to clip up the corners of the sheets. I saw this technique on a Youtube video as well and it worked great. This meant I could only use 4 of the 9 shelves since the clipped sheets were taller but I didn't need more than 3 trays for each dinner per night.

Research

I also did a ton of research online for dehydrating food, how to do it and what worked best. Many of the websites for back packing were about bulk dehydrated foods and adding them together to make different combinations like dried potato flakes, bacon bits and chives. I needed a protein base for most of my meals so I had to get creative. The sodium content was really bad for many of the bulk dried products. I wanted to make the food I like at home and take that with me. I cannot say enough about one website I went to over and over again. www.backpackingchef.com. He is amazing and has everything written down into details!

- Let me make a quick note here. There are a ton of websites and blogs that have healthy alternatives for hiking and back packing food. I do not want to in anyway disparage the group as a whole. I got so many great suggestions from blogs and websites. It all came together for my menu and trip. Find what you need and use that, one way or another is not wrong or right, this is just how I did it.

Reading about dehydrating proteins I learned that you need lean meats and there were specific types of meat that would not work. So I planned my meals using ground meats. Later in the recipe section I will talk about prep for the ground meats.

Variety is the spice of life. This is true when you are in the middle of nowhere with a long way to go. I wanted to not only have food I liked but different flavors I could count on to be interesting. I wanted the food to be nutritious and healthy as well. We were going to be rowing a lot of the way so we needed energy to burn.

We did also have plenty of oatmeal and other rehydrated foods on board so we could eat breakfast whenever we wanted. I tried to get dehydrated eggs but they were just not good in my opinion.

Notes:

The Food Prep

My go-to foods are things like chili, spaghetti, curry stews etc. I set out to try to dehydrate a whole meal every night. I would make double batch of something for dinner in and then spread half of it out on the sheets and dehydrate overnight. It was fun to think up the next day's meal. Keep in mind I am adding recipes here exactly how I did them but you can use gluten products instead of the gluten free stuff I used. It will be the same.

I worked on having a variety of foods as well as adding as much nutrition as I could. When I could I threw in ground flax seeds, veggies and tried to keep the food as whole as possible.

It is important to cut the food you are going to cook into consistent sizes. If you have pieces that are bigger they will take longer to rehydrate. Try to keep everything similar shapes and sizes.

Some folks worried about the meat being in a warm environment. We stored the dehydrated packets at the water line so it was never warmer than 34 degrees Fahrenheit. I would not be worried about the

dehydrated meat if it was warmer, with the vacuum

packaging the risk of it going bad is minimal to none because there is no oxygen added until it is cut open and we are in a very cold climate.

If you were going to be in warm or hot weather I would keep it dehydrated for 1 week and feel fine about it. Use your own discretion when making these decisions.

Now you have the basics, add your own favorite recipes to the list and do not worry about trying something out. Almost everything will rehydrate wonderfully if you started out with something tasty. Remember a few simple rules. Lean meats are necessary, fat does not dehydrate. Ground meats work best. Add bread crumbs to your ground meats.

Portioning out the food is a little trickier, soups dehydrate down more than chili or thicker sauces. I would add about one solid packed cup or cup and a half of dehydrated food to each sealed packet as the water will make it double in size.

The containers for rehydrating we used were 16 oz so

one cup is 8 oz and the rehydrated water would bring it up close to 16 oz when I is done. The only one different was the chicken noodle soup I made which needed a little less as it was supposed to be a broth.

Snacks

Snacks are a big part of motivation when doing a race like the Transpac or R2AK. We did buy the usual chocolates, nuts and crunchy stuff. We each had our own bag of snacks so when we were on watch we knew we had something to keep us awake up on deck. These were all bagged separate so we could grab them as we went up on watch so we didn't wake anyone trying to get snacks. My biggest personal concern was my diet avoids high salt, sugar and wheat so a lot of the ready-made snacks were not good for me. So I worked on getting good snacks I could eat that tasted good.

I added some beef jerky, nuts and raisins in packs and anything that was more of a whole food nature. Trader Joe's has a great pre-packaged selection of nuts, seeds and raisins that work well for this type of trip. I also had a bag of dehydrated yogurt that was great protein and whole fruit so that helped a lot, I have included the recipe for that in the next section.

Small bags of chips are a great go to as well. I eat pretty

healthy but nothing works to keep me awake like a small bag of Doritos or cheese puffs. Bigger bags might get soggy and chewy quickly. Be creative and remember that an indulgence can go a long way for snacks.

A friend of the team created individual bags for each of us as a farewell gift. In each of the over-sized zip lock bags was chips, candy, gum etc. I think the chips are a big hit in small bags because you lack crunch when you are out there for a long time. Also a lot of my food was lower salt so a little bit was great.

Notes:

⛵Chapter 6

Recipes for Dehydrating

I included these recipes that I made myself at home. These fit easily into 3 or 4 sheets inside the dehydrator.

Be creative, think of meals you really like, what makes you think yum, I want to eat that again? Ask team mates what they like to eat. Have each teammate make a big pot of their favorite food and dehydrate that for the team. Keep it interesting, share the work and get everyone involved. It all helps with comradery.

Spaghetti with ground beef (dehydrator on 145 degrees for 8-12 hours)

3 lbs. of ground beef

1 tbsp of olive oil

1 ½ cups of gluten free bread crumbs

4 green zucchinis diced

¼ cup of ground flax seeds

1 medium yellow onion diced

4 cloves of garlic diced

10 ounces of mushrooms (1 container) diced

3 jars of spaghetti sauce

1 can of diced tomatoes

1 package of gluten free spaghetti noodles

Dehydrated ground meat can be very tough and will not rehydrate easily. The Backpacking Chef taught me to use bread crumbs to help it rehydrate. It really works! Take the ground beef and massage the bread crumbs into it, thank you backpacking chef! Then they will rehydrate and make the meat soft.

After the meat is all breaded up add the olive oil to the pan and then the add all of the veggies, cook them for about 5 minutes and then add the meat, brown it up and then add the flax seed, sauce and tomatoes.

Let this come to a boil and then turn the heat down and cook for about 15 minutes, this will allow the sauce to mix together better. Turn it off, add your cooked spaghetti, as little or as much as you desire, and stir together. Take the whole mess over to the dehydrator and pour 1/4 to 1/3 of it on each sheet. You want to make sure it is not too thick, this will take a lot longer to dehydrate.

I then turned on the dehydrator and let it dehydrate overnight. Something as thick as a spaghetti is going to take 8-12 hours at 145 degrees. I also found that I needed to "stir" the food. I would pick it up and move it around and flip it over. This helped get it dried all the way through. It is going to look awful. You will think there is no way that stuff is going to be edible but believe me it will soak up hot water and be delicious when you need it to be. Break it up into 1 ½ cup portions and put into vacuum sealed bags or zip top bags for storage. Write the name of the food on the bag so when it is time to reheat you know what you are getting.

Chili (145 degrees, 8-12 hours)

1 lb. ground turkey

1 lb. ground pork

1 cup of bread crumbs

1 green bell pepper chopped

1 red bell pepper chopped

2 stalks of celery chopped

1 medium to large onion chopped

4 cloves of garlic chopped

2 tbsp. chili powder

1 tsp. cumin

½ tsp oregano

½ tsp. cayenne pepper (more if you like it hotter)

½ tsp. black pepper

(4) 14.5 oz cans of tomato sauce

(2) 14.5 oz. cans of chopped tomatoes

1 small can of tomato paste

1 tbs. olive oil

Massage bread crumbs into both pounds of meat. You can choose any type of ground meat to your tastes. Heat olive oil in a pan, add chopped vegetables and garlic, sauté until slightly tender, add ground meats and fry. You can let the edges get crispy on the meat as this can add flavor. Add spices while you are cooking the meat.

Once it is cooked and broken down into smaller sized pieces add all the sauces and tomatoes. Add paste and stir. Let simmer for 20 minutes and then let it cool down. Pour chili onto three trays for the dehydrator using the binder clip method to keep the liquid in the trays.

Dehydrate 8-12 hours at 145 degrees, stirring and turning over the chili until it is completely dry. Break up the chili into meal size amounts, about 1 ½ cups, then seal with a vacuum sealer or zip the top of the baggy being used. Write the name on the bag so when it is time to eat you know what you are getting.

West African Ground Nut Stew (145 degrees, 8-12 hours)

I love this stew anytime. I thought the healthy combination of veggies, tomato and peanut butter would be welcome out on the water. It is also vegan so, there's that.

1 Tbsp of olive oil

1 medium Onion Diced

1 yellow or red pepper diced

2 cloves of garlic minced

2 tsps of minced ginger

2 jalapenos, seeded and diced

2 cups of water

2 cups of tomato juice

14 ounces stewed tomatoes

2 cups of diced sweet potatoes

1 Tbsp of dried parsley

1 ½ tsps dried thyme

1 ½ tsps. Cumin

½ tsp salt

½ cup chunky peanut butter

2 cups of Swiss Chard cut into small pieces

Heat the oil and add onion, garlic, ginger. Sauté these together for around 4 minutes then stir in water, tomato juice, sweet potatoes and seasonings.

Cook for 25 minutes then add peanut butter and stir in well.

Add the Swiss chard and simmer an additional 5-10 minutes. Take off the heat and let cool. Pour 1/3 of the contents onto one of the non-stick sheets with the binder clips on them. Take all 3 sheets and trays and put them into the dehydrator. Dehydrate for 8-12 hours at 145 degrees, stirring and flipping contents until they are completely dry. Add 1 ½ cups of dried material to a vacuum seal bag or zip top bag. Write the name of the contents on the bag for future use.

Curry Chicken Salad Snack

This was a taste packed addition to the snacks. It did require hot water and sitting for a little bit but was different from chips and nuts. I came across this recipe and substituted canned chicken meat because it dehydrates really well. We also had snack crackers on the boat so this went perfect with those.

4 cans of chicken meat, 4.5 ounces

1 ¼ cups mayonnaise

1 1/2 tsps of curry powder

1/8 tsp of ground ginger

Salt and pepper to taste

1 stalk of celery with all the strings pulled off of it and diced small

2 Tbps of raisins

1/4 cup of chives

Shred up the chicken and add all of the other ingredients. Spread this out into a tray for the dehydrator and run the machine for 8 hours, stirring and flipping the contents as needed. When it's done take 1 cup of the mix and add it to a vacuum seal bag or zip top bag for storing. Additions can include apples diced small, cashews, cranberries. Be creative!

Yogurt roll ups (125 degrees, 4-8 hours)

I did a little research on how to make some more high protein snacks and came across some videos that showed how to dehydrate full fat yogurt. It would come out soft enough to chew but maintain all of its probiotic properties as well. There are a ton of combinations you can use for this too.

1 cup of full fat yogurt

½ - ¾ cup of fresh or frozen berries

Add a sweetener if you are not used to tart yogurt, stevia, honey, sugar

Additional adds – ground flax seed, cinnamon, vanilla, chocolate, the sky is the limit!

Blend together. On your non-stick sheets add a layer of parchment paper, this will hold the yogurt together for easy eating. Spread out the yogurt until it is about the same thickness, ¼ inch, across the parchment. Put trays into the dehydrator at 125 degrees for 4-8 hours. After it is dry you can then roll it up and then slice the parchment into 6-8 individual rolls. These easily go into zip top bags and can withstand room temperature storage as well as getting beat up a little bit. If you do not store it on parchment paper it tends to clump together and is more difficult to eat. These were great treats in the snack bag, lots of flavor and chewy, definitely kept me awake on the inside passage.

Breakfast bags

I went to a bulk food store and bought powdered milk. Then I purchased cereal with different flavors. Once I added the powdered milk it was ready to go with just some water added. You can do this with the granola recipe I have on here. I also added freeze dried raspberries and blueberries for a little added zing and some vitamin C. Get creative. If you can eat it for breakfast you can add powdered milk and take it in a baggy for whenever you need something fun to eat. I'm thinking captain crunch, cocoa puffs, anything with crunch is appreciated when you are out there. You can also pre-pack your own oatmeal mixes and cut down on some of the salt that comes with the pre-packed oatmeal from the store.

Really Yummy Homemade Granola (not dehydrated), from my friend Nancy Morrison!

This is a surprisingly flexible recipe. Add as many nuts as you like, dried fruits, mix it up. Bake it a little longer if you like it crispier. It's all up to you. Once it has dried you can add it to your baggies with a little powered milk.

Dry mix:

6 Cups of Oats

1-2 cups of walnuts or other nuts

1 cup of sunflower seeds

2-3 cups shredded coconut

Wet mix:

¾ cup of coconut oil

¾ cup maple syrup or brown sugar

½ cup of brown sugar

1 tsp of vanilla

1 Tbsp of Cinnamon

2 tsp of salt

Blend these together and spread out on parchment paper or silicon sheet and bake at 300 degrees for 10 minutes, stir and bake an additional 10 minutes.

This next section covers the

Trans Pac Race I cooked for in 2011

⛵Chapter 7

Creating frozen meals for the Trans Pac

This section of the book covers meal prep for an ocean race when you have more space and equipment to hold and cook food, I wrote it before I raced on the R2AK.

The original content:

The not quite complete guide to one woman's search to feed her man (and a few others) on the Trans Pac 2011 (and then on the R2AK), imperfect but there you have it! I have also added a new section on dehydrating food for long passages and races. I did this for our team of 4 women who raced the R2AK or Race to Alaska in 2017. Unlike the frozen pans of food we had to be aware of weight and took dehydrated food along. I have started that section in the second half of the book.

This is a quick reference guide to what worked for me. Let me add a disclaimer right here and now, I am not a master cook, sailor, organizer or anything even bordering on professional. The crew said they liked it and no one threw things at me when they got to Hawaii. The goal here was to finish a task I happily accepted before really knowing what it entailed.

There are FAR greater experts and a great many better novices than me. I just never found info on line to help me when I was preparing so I thought I would fling it out there in case someone found themselves in my situation.

So, you may need to prepare foods for a race or a long sailing trip. Here is some info for you to think about. There are a ton of things to take into consideration. I hope to have listed my observations here. This is absolutely not what others have done, just what I have gleaned from websites, blogs, message boards, friends and now experience.

Here are the 7 Main Categories I worked with for the Trans Pac, if you have more God bless you and good luck! I wanted to review what I had to think about when planning for the Trans Pacific Race.

1. The Owner
2. The Galley
3. The Crew
4. The Trip
5. The Food
6. Organizing for the Race and Crew
7. Recipes

It was a lot of fun finding out I could do this on my own. Of course I had my taste testers, Mark and Amanda who helped a lot, trial and error on the recipes and everyone's kind words when I got there.

I hope you find the experience as fun and rewarding as I did. The best reward for the cook is being there when the boat comes in!!!!

Stephanie

If you need to get a hold of me just email me at slyohio@hotmail.com.

Chapter 8

Trans Pac: The Owner

I was extraordinarily lucky to be working with a couple who wanted their crew to have the best and that included the quality of food and experience. I was actually following in the footsteps of the first mate and wife of the boat owner. She had provisioned for the Pacific Cup Race the year before and sailed on the boat as well, what a woman. There was an amazing collection of foods, exotic, tasty and I hear just great, that she served up for that race.

They weren't so lucky this time, I am a simple cook and I was not going on board which told me I could make what I wanted and not hear them complain in real time. Their past chef was instrumental in helping me get my arms around the task. The difference this trip was the first mate was not going along so it would be up to the crew and boat owner to handle the food while underway. The owner said "Do whatever you have to and I will help out when I am on board".

So, it is up to the owner to dictate what kind of food comes on board and is the first consideration when making preparations. You will work hand in hand with the owner, the crew and what their expectations are for the preparation of the food when creating the menu.

Here is a list of things to start you on your way in communicating with the owner.

1. **Expense Limit –**
   What is the budget for the food? This is figured out in a lot of different ways. If you are provisioning for an owner and they give you a budget limit that is one thing. If you are splitting the dishes between different members of the crew then it is up to each person to carry the expense for their dish, with considerations for weight etc. (see food section for other food specifications). If you are taking on the expense yourself then you have a lot of choices. Food can be very expensive or super cheap or in the middle; it all depends on who is cooking it and the quality of the ingredients.

   Create a budget for yourself if you are creating the dishes or suggest a budget for those who are adding dishes to the menu along the way.

This budget also needs to take into account snacks and extras. You can divide a budget up for each of the days and then for each of the meals to see where you may end up. I have some recommendations below to help you out. As I say a lot, it all depends on the owner, organizer and cook as to how money is spent and where you can splurge.

We had 9 crew members going on the race and the calculated amount of days they would be at sea was 10. So I needed to make three meals a day as well as two types of snacks for that day. I chose to create all the meals from scratch which cost a little more money than a prepackaged meal plan would.

2. **Dry foods or Frozen –**
   Find out from the captain/owner what his expectations are. Some of the fastest race boats have only freeze dried meals on board. They can save on time and most have a high calorie content. These are not always morale boosting choices but if you are on a serious race boat and that is the food, you eat it.

We were lucky enough to have a frozen option. The freezer on board the sailboat could accommodate some of the meals for the later part of the trip. I opted to make all the meals frozen for the time frame we were given but the owner also decided to have some dry meals on board for emergency. The meals that did not fit into the freezer that was on board the boat were packed into larger separate coolers. These would be the first meals eaten. When I followed the races online I noticed there were boats that came across difficulties, broken parts etc., and they had to be at sea longer than planned for. That means planning ahead for any possible delays and adding on freeze dried foods just in case.

Make sure your meal plan takes into account how much room you have for frozen meals and how many freeze dried meals you will need to supply as well.

3. **Weight considerations –**
   This will also depend on the expectation of the boat owner, what style of boat, speed, competition. Is there a weight limit? This is a great

question for the captain/owner. Even if there are weight considerations freeze dried food is going to require water for hydration so there is weight involved in the food no matter what.

4. **Do they care?** –

   Some people don't care as much. Of course you are frequently in a race to win, you hope, but the quality of food and the breaks they provide are often much needed respite from the trials of the race and a good captain wants morale to be high! Find out from your crew if they have any specifics they would like to see, cravings, needs and wants. It is fun to fit in meals they can look forward to.

⛵Chapter 9

Trans Pac: The Galley

Some race boats do not have a galley, they don't even have a bathroom, they have a bucket and a burner. This is not their book. They could use some of the recipes if they want to and lash everything down in some coolers. When preparing for the trip it is most important to know exactly what is on the boat as far as space for storage, space for cooking, equipment for cooking and equipment for eating.

Every boat has a different galley or lack thereof. The more competitive boats have a burner and that is where you heat up the water in order to hydrate the dry foods. If this is the case then you only need to measure where the dry foods are going to be and how they can be easily accessed. If there will be more cooking than this you will need to see where the frozen/refrigerated goods go as well as dried goods, snacks and other material needs for the meals.

1. **Dry Good Storage –**
   There are some really creative places to keep food. Go over the boat with the captain/owner and ask to see all the cubby holes available.

Ask if they will be used for anything and if so what. Look into the walls, table tops; small niches are perfect for bite size candy bars or snack bars. Feel free to really dig. Often these little spaces cannot be used for sailing, their too small, but are perfect to shove a small bag of goodies. These are a life saver in the middle of the race. Much of the dry good storage I used was on the top rail bunk that would not be needed for a sleeping sailor.

2. **Fridge –**
   This is going to be a critical measurement. You want to see what space you have for refrigeration because this is going to be the only room to work with for your fresh fruits, vegetables and any other immediate use foods. So get in there with a measuring tape and get the length, width and height. When it comes time to compile everything you are sending you will want to know the fresh foods you buy will fit in here.

3. **Freezer –** This is going to be critical as well. Often a boat has either a freezer or a fridge. I was lucky because ours had both.

However, the freezer could not hold the 10-11 days' worth of food required for the trip so I had to know what I could fit in and what I needed to find more room for. Measure the length, width and height here as well. If you do not have a freezer there are alternatives.

Additional frozen meals were placed in coolers and taped shut. Then they were taken to a commercial facility, any restaurant or food supplier will do, where we attempted to drop their core temperature as low as possible before loading them aboard.

4. **Snack Spots** – This goes back to the little spaces, cubbies and walls. I was lucky enough to have some great hiding spots in the middle of the boat where the drop leaves of the table went down. There were lift out boards and most of our snacks fit in there. Also along the walls were edges and things to bungee bags to. We had a lot of room. Trouble was not packing too much! Having a variety of easy to grab and tasty snacks can make a bad day better, keep this in mind when buying snacks, nutritious, yummy, spicy, sweet and salty are all key.

5. **Oven and stove tops –**

   Just as critical as the food is the place to cook it. Make sure you get measurements for the oven if there is one. You will definitely need to have this for the baking pans if you plan to prepare food or freeze it and have the crew cook it up later on. My experience has been there are about 3000, I exaggerate, kinds of pans and some will not fit. It would be horrible to look forward to a meal and not be able to heat it up.

   Our oven measurements were 13.5 inches deep by 16 inches wide and 9 inches high so I found pans that would fit in there.

   Find out whether the crew has a pan to cook in on the stove top and what the expectation will be for them to cook, sauce pan, fry pan or a big pot. Most of my meals were put into the oven to heat up but I did make a soup and a few stove top things. They had a big pan to boil in and the stove could accommodate the large wave action. It is a good idea to ensure that the stove works, there is a large pan to work with and the crew is capable of cooking. If not then all of your larger meals need to be in pans for the oven.

6. Equipment

This is just as critical as well. Ask the captain/owner where all the equipment is. Dig through drawers if you have to. Find the utensils, bowls, pans and everything else that is available. As the food preparer it is your job to figure out what they will cook with, on and in as well as what they will put the food in and what they will eat it with.

Pans:

Oven - If you are cooking food to be reheated or baked then you will want to get pans that fit in the oven. Obviously use the measurements you have taken from before and purchase the correct aluminum pans from a store that fit those specifications. These will probably be aluminum due to weight constraints as well as purchase price. It is a great idea to have one hard pan to slip these aluminum pans into for use in the oven. The aluminum pans get flimsy when they are thawing and reheating so the hard pan really helps a lot. You can buy the hard pan at a restaurant supply store and they can use it over and over again.

Stove top- One large pot can be used for so much. We had one to heat up water for spaghetti and soup. If someone is cooking on the trip you might be able to use a fry pan but most of the food should be cooked ahead of time.

Plates, Bowls and Silver Wear

Bowls-Don't laugh but they found out on the trip before mine that nothing works as well as dog food bowls for eating at sea. The smaller sized bowls often have grippy strips on the bottom, they are deep and can handle a lot of food. In rough seas when you have been up taking care of things having an easy to use bowl is a life saver.

Utensils – You will need obviously spoons, enough to last the trip as well as a big spoon to serve out of the containers.

Make sure there are enough utensils for them to use with the baked dishes.

Plates – Most of the eating would be out of the dog food bowls but a nice supply of paper plates also helps with a quick sandwich. Make sure you have a supply of these as well.

Chapter 10

Trans Pac: The Crew

Find out about your crew and any special needs they may have. I found out by talking to my crew that they had a concern for constipation. They didn't want to be stuck at sea and worry about this. So I worked fiber into my recipes, bought Prune juice and would advise anyone stocking a boat to do the same.

1. How many – This will obviously have the biggest impact on how much you make. I always tried to figure about 1 ½ times a normal serving times the number of crew. They can always toss whatever is left over out. Making too much is also a bad thing as added weight is a no no on a racing sailboat.

2. Allergies – Luckily I didn't have anyone with allergies. If you have some tough allergies I would probably advise that person to bring their own rations, you would not want someone to deal with a huge allergic reaction far from land. Otherwise I tried to cook things that were pretty basic.

3. Preferences – Be careful what you wish for on this. I love to take suggestions but if you open the door too far then you are being dictated too about everything they want. I liked to ask just so I included them in some of the decisions.

4. Cook- Is someone in charge of the cooking or will that person change throughout the trip? Our boat had different crew members who cooked throughout the trip. I have met other people who go on these long trips just to provide the food for the crew, lucky them, and that works out great. On my trip the crew was not going to be allocating a crew member so I needed to have very simple step by step instructions laid out for the crew members to

5. heat the food and what dry goods were meant to go with it. I will share how I did that later on. Find out if there is a crew member who will be designated per shift for heating and feeding their shift members.

⛵ Chapter 11

Trans Pac: The Trip

Where the trip is headed is a big deal. What will the temperatures be, could it be rough, how long and the purpose. So much can go into the planning when you take into account the seas and temperatures. Some cooks say it doesn't matter, get the food on the boat, they will eat it if they are hungry. This is very true, hungry sailors will eat what you feed them. So number of days and intensity are the main concerns for the trip portion of planning.

1. **How Many Days** – Of course the number of days they will be at sea is the biggest portion of the planning. That number can vary widely so you will want to ask around and find out what the shortest and longest version of their trip would be. In our case the sailboat did the Pacific Cup in just 9 days when they were planning for 12 and then the Trans Pac in 11 when we planned for 10. I got lucky, the cooked meals ran out as they got to shore, just crumbs and dry meals left.

Calculate the average days it will take and add a meal or two. Dry food, as unappetizing as it may sound can fill in any extra time.

2. **Purpose, race, cruise, combo** – If this is a serious race then the food needs to be nutritious, easy to heat and eat and quick clean up. If it is a cruise then you can plan for more layers to the meals. You could even have a first course in small pans and side dishes in separate pans. If you are that good then go for it. I planned most of the meals for a serious sailboat race and that is mostly what this book is about. There may have to be another book for the cruising long distance cook!

3. **Weather changes, going from cold to hot** – This is also another section that you may not need to worry about. I thought through the menu to make dishes that were gentle on the stomach the first day and then easier to eat in warmer weather on the last day as they came into Hawaii. Some folks will say just put the food out and it will get eaten. You can see some of the recipes at the end of the book.

⛵Chapter 12

Trans Pac: The Food

I don't know about you but most folks I know love their food. It was important to me that I cooked dishes I would like to eat. It didn't come out that way always but I did shoot for tasty and easy to heat.

What I took into consideration when planning the food and snacks was morale. I learned a lot after the race and would change things up more for future cooking but keep in mind when they are exhausted it is the food that they most look forward to.

1. **Frozen or freeze dried** – There are a lot of choices when it comes to dried food these days. Even if you are faced with this as your choice it can be picked out and varied according to all the great companies that

   package the newest dried foods. If you are in charge of the water for the food make sure you get enough.

Frozen food that you create yourself has the best variety available and you can get really creative by going online and looking up recipes for different meals and combinations.

2. **Portions, crew size** – Sailboat crews get HUNGRY! I am not sure I made enough for them all and knowing what I know now I would have tried to make more per person. I stated before try to make about 1 ½ portions per person of each meal. Most recipes list portions in the recipe itself. If you wonder how much you need go to a sports bar during a sporting event and watch these guys eat. That's about how much you need, our crew burns upwards of 5000 calories a day, or more.

3. **Nutrition** – I tried to balance nutrition in most of the recipes. I ground up vegetables and added fiber powder whenever I could. If it was a tomato base I added broccoli and green beans and ground it up. Think about how you could make it as balanced with fats, fiber and carbs so they feel full and well fed.

4. **Fresh food, fruits and veggies** – We sent as many fresh vegetables and fruits as we could on the trip. They last a little while so it seemed to work for the first week. I also created some frozen vegetable dishes that were easy to heat up. Add vegetables to as many meals as possible.

   - Types of vegetables to have on the boat would be salad mixes in the bag, pre-cut veggies, salads, a large watermelon keeps great for later in the trip. Apples and oranges can keep well outside of the fridge, just secure them well and let the crew know they are there.

5. **Fiber** – I used a fiber power in my less fibrous dishes, it is a tasteless and clear powder that is undetectable. I used a brand called Sprinkle Fiber. It was a flavor free table fiber that I found no one noticed at home. If that seems like too much then there are alternatives. My crew was concerned about fiber so I bought some prune juice. I would also include three bottles of prune juice so there is plenty as well as snack packs of prunes and raisins.

You could even send or recommend they buy fiber pills. These are so easy to take these days and could help the crew out.

6. **Snacks** – I found out these were very, very important. In between meals a snack bar or chocolate treat is just what you need. I bought candy bars, granola bars and lots of different things but I would probably have bought a larger variety so it broke up the monotony. I think it would have been fun for a new type of snack to come out around day 4, then again on day 7. You can't plan for snacks quite the same way you plan for meals so think about each crew member and plan 5 snacks per day of different sizes, small candy, nutrition bar and nuts and seeds. You can buy big containers of nuts they can store in the side cupboard as well. Keep in mind lots of extra bread and peanut butter and jelly is a huge favorite. They can run out of peanut butter fast so stock up.

7. **Half Way Meal** – This is a huge tradition on many of the boats. On the trip before mine the owner's wife cooked an amazing meal with

Filet mignon and more. I didn't know how much effort they were going to be able to put in for this meal and I tried to plan for it as best I could. Depending on the race, weather, wind and boat health the half way could be hard to predict. It is a really fun time for the crew to celebrate.

8. **Coffee/Tea-** This is all about preference and is a good conversation to have with the crew. How will they be making coffee? How strong do they like it? What flavors do they like? Do they want tea? How will they heat the water? Caffeine is such an important part of the shift change and critical to the crew. Once you find out preferences calculate out how much you will need for everyone for the longer version of the trip and then add one more bag. This should be ground up and available to them to just throw in and make. Plan out sugar and milk for the coffee as well. This will go into the fridge for ongoing use. Have some dry milk as backup.

9. **Surprises** – When you are living through
   pounding waves, sleep deprivation, and lord
   knows what else it is an amazing thing to have
   great things to eat, crunchy, salty sweet treats
   and small surprises. Many loved ones pack a
   letter or surprise gift for the half way mark.
   Others pack treats in their luggage as a
   surprise. As the cook you can pack a surprise
   anywhere along the way. Put it in between
   other meals, add something special and just
   think of things you might want if you were
   hungry, tired and far from home.

⛵Chapter 13

Trans Pac: Organizing

Since there was no cook per say on the trip I needed to create a well-organized system for the crew to use when it was their turn to cook dinner. I created a menu that detailed what needed to be used for that meal and what needed to be prepped for the next one.

I then laminated it and put it in a binder that would fit easily in a cubby in the galley so they could just open up to the next page and use the directions.

1. **Menu** – I listed out the menu in blocked squares for breakfast, lunch and dinner so they knew what to look for. Then I created detailed instructions for that meal in the planner book. This way the crew had a snapshot of what each meal was going to be and could also go into the more detailed book if they were in charge of heating it up.

I created the entire menu in an excel spreadsheet that fit on two pages. Having the spreadsheet also helped me stack the foods as I packed them.

2. **Instructions** – The instructions were as clear as possible, detailing what they should be heating that day. I also wrote the name of the meal on top of the container with that food in it. So the instructions might say:

_____

Day 6
Breakfast: Oatmeal, cereal, bars

Lunch:
Manwich and lunch meats
Use leftover French rolls and bread

Dinner:
Heat Beef and Rice Casserole in oven.

For next Day:
(Take Pork and Potatoes, in pan, and spaghetti, garlic bread, in bags, out of freezer)

_____

They knew what to look for from the freezer and what to use out of the dry bags. There were also instructions for the next day's meals.

3. **Binder** – The Binder came in really handy to keep the instructions in one place. If you can find a place to store it on board out of the way great. I would laminate it, punch a hole through the corner and use one of those key ring clasps to hook it to the galley if you don't have a cubby.

4. **Organization** – Once you know your menu and have everything bought you want to stack it backwards, so the last meals to be eaten are on the bottom and the first ones are on the top. You then want to get the bags, paper or recyclable, that you will use for dry goods like bread, rolls, spaghetti etc. and stack those backwards too. If Salsa and Chips are the last day they might go in the last dry goods bag. If you have 8 dry goods bags then the salsa and

chips would be in bag 8. If you have 10 days you could even label the dry good bags according to the day it should be used, Day 10 on back through Day 1. Make sure your instructions tell them what bag to look for during that meal. It helps them out a lot.

Chapter 14

Menu Set Up

Here is the fun part, get creative. I am sharing some of the recipes I used but make things you really like. I pre-cooked all the meals for the crew before freezing them. The casseroles I left a little under cooked so they would reheat with some moisture still left in them.

Here is the detailed menu with instructions that I used. I am adding it here exactly how I had it in the binder.

Day 1

Lunch:

Fresh sandwiches

Dinner:

Chicken and Rice, In refrigerator, not frozen.

In bags, heat up in oven or stovetop

Day 2

Breakfast:

Hot oats, bars and cereal

Lunch:

Lunch meats or peanut butter

Dinner:

BBQ pork sandwiches

Pork is stored in fridge, heat in pan

French Bread Hoagie Rolls in

Dry storage area

Frozen Corn, needs to be cooked on the stovetop, add one stick of butter as you heat it up, three bags in freezer.

For Next day: (Take the Chili, in bags, and breakfast burritos, (smaller ones in bags) out of the freezer)

Day 3

Breakfast:

Hot oats, cereal, bars

Lunch:

Lunch meat/ peanut butter

Dinner:

Chili, in bags, heat on stove top

Toppings for chili, in fridge:

Shredded cheese (Mexican)

Baggy of chives, freezer

Tub of sour cream, fridge, Tortilla Chips

Bagged Salad is also available in fridge

For Next day:

(Take Franks and Beans out of freezer)

Day 4

Breakfast:

Breakfast Burritos, two kinds, mild and hot

Lunch:

Lunch meat/peanut butter

Dinner: Franks and Beans,

Bagged Salad in fridge

For next Day:

(Take out Half Way meal, roast beef in bags, Mushrooms, Baked Potato casserole, green beans in a bag)

Day 5: Half Way!

Breakfast:

Oatmeal, cereal bars

Lunch:

Lunch Meat/ Peanut Butter

Dinner:

Half Way Meal

Stuffed mushrooms are an appetizer, cook them

in the stove first.

Heat roast on stove top and potatoes in oven.

Heat garlic green beans last.

For next Day:

(Take Manwich and Lasagna, and breakfast casserole

out of the freezer)

Day 6

Breakfast: Oatmeal, cereal, bars

Lunch:

Manwich and lunch meats

Use leftover French rolls and bread

Dinner:

Heat Lasagna in oven.

For next Day:

(Take Beef and Rice Casserole, in pan, and spaghetti, garlic bread, in bags, out of freezer)

Day 7

Breakfast: Breakfast casserole, heat in oven.

Lunch:

Lunch meats/ peanut butter

Dinner:

Beef and Rice casserole, heat in oven

Day 8

Breakfast:

Oatmeal, cereal, bars

Lunch: Lunch meat/peanut butter

Dinner:

Spaghetti and Garlic Bread:

Heat up Garlic bread in oven.

Boil noodles on stove top, after they are drained

empty sauce on top of them and serve, small shaker

of Parmesan in dry goods storage.

For next Day:

(Take larger Burritos out of freezer)

Day 9

Breakfast:

Oatmeal, cereal and bars

Lunch:

Lunch meat, peanut butter

Dinner:

Burritos, heat in oven

Two types, mild ground beef taco flavor and

Barbacoa, spicy flavorful shredded beef.

Salsa and chip in dry good area.

For next day:

(Take Chicken soup out of freezer, in bags)

Day 10

Breakfast:

Oatmeal, cereal, bars

Lunch:

Lunch Meat, peanut butter

Dinner:

Chicken Tortilla Soup

Heat bags on stove top

Use last of sour cream, leftover shredded cheese, leftover chives and tortilla chips.

(Hopefully you get in before this! After this you are on to the rest of the snacks and freeze dried food.)

I have also included some of the recipes for the meals I cooked.

⛵ Chapter 15

Recipes

Day 1: Chicken and Rice (First Day meal for any upset tummies)

4 Lbs. of boneless skinless chicken thighs

Soaked overnight in Teriyaki sauce

Grilled until cooked through

Cooled and chopped into bite size pieces

Stir Fried rice

4-8 green onions chopped, to taste

8 large eggs

4 tsp. salt and pepper

8 cups cooked rice

4-6 Tbsp. Soy sauce

2 cups thin shredded cabbage

1 cup thin shredded carrots

Cooked peas, frozen is best

4 tbsp. of oil

Lightly beat eggs and set aside

Heat oil in a wok type pan or a large skillet that can fit all the ingredients.

Add all of the veggies and cook until tender.

Remove veggies. Cook eggs in the same pan using a light scramble until just done, remove and clean pan.

Heat additional 2 tbsp. oil and add rice. Break apart as it heats so the grains separate. Add Soy, veggies and egg. Stir well and take off heat. Add green onions and chicken. Serve.

Day 2: The BBQ pork eaten on day 2 was Trader Joes pulled pork sandwich meat. They had eaten it on the last race and really liked it.

Day 3: Chili, I make different versions all the time.

Chili with beans

1 lb. ground beef

1 lb. ground pork

1 green bell pepper chopped

1 red bell pepper chopped

2 stalks of celery chopped

1 medium to large onion chopped

4 cloves of garlic chopped

2 tbsp. chili powder

1 tsp. cumin

½ tsp oregano

½ tsp. cayenne pepper (more if you like it hotter)

½ tsp. black pepper

(4) 14.5 oz cans of tomato sauce

(2) 14.5 oz. cans of chopped tomatoes

1 small can of tomato paste

1 14.5 oz can of red kidney beans

1 14.5 oz. can of light kidney beans

1 tbs. olive oil

Heat olive oil in a pan, add chopped vegetables and garlic, sauté until slightly tender, add ground meats and fry. You can let the edges get crispy on the meat as this can add flavor. Add spices while you are cooking the meat. Once it is cooked and chopped into bite size pieces add all the sauces and tomatoes. Add paste and stir. Then add both cans of beans. Let simmer for 20 minutes and then let it cool down. I put this into two gallon Ziploc bags, double bagged, and froze it flat. It saved a lot of space this way.

Breakfast Burritos

1 14.5 oz. can refried beans

18 eggs

1 mild and 1 hot package of ground breakfast sausage, cooked and crumbled

Sour cream

Shredded cheese

1 onion chopped

1 green bell pepper

1 tbsp. olive oil

Flour tortillas, smaller size

Hot salsa

Mild salsa

Cook the eggs as a large batch of scrambled eggs. Heat oil in a pan and cook the onion and pepper. Heat up the beans in a pan and work until smooth.

Put out all materials on counter and start assembling the burritos. Make sure you separate out the mild and hot. Wrap in aluminum foil and label hot or mild.

These can all be heated in one large pan in the oven and then grab and unwrap and eat.

Franks and Beans (super simple meal)

3 packages of Johnsonville Original Bratwurst (15 brats)

8 large cans, 28 oz. Bush's Vegetarian baked beans

Cook the brats on a grill. Get them charred outside, this adds a lot of flavor.

Pour the beans into the pan you will be freezing them in.

Slice the brats into 1 inch wide pieces and then stir into beans.

Slow Roasted Beef – Another very easy to cook meal

6 lbs. of beef roast

½ cup of flour

4 onions, sliced

3 tbsp. olive oil

Salt and pepper to taste

Another ½ cup of flour

3 tbsp. of butter

Cut roast into large chunks. Coat with the flour and salt and pepper all sides.

Heat oil in a pan and add the roast pieces to it. Brown as well as you can on all sides. Places onion slices on bottom of slow cooker then add roast pieces as they get browned.

Turn on high for ½ hour, then low for 6 hours.

After you finish roasting the meat take it out of the slow cooker. In a sauce pan melt the butter and add the flour. Cook it until it gets a little bubbly. Slowly add the juice from the slow cooker and stir thoroughly. Continue until all of the juice has been added to the gravy mixture. Break up the beef in the pan you will be freezing it in and pour the gravy over it. I used a smaller pan for this.

Garlic Green Beans

I prefer to use fresh green beans for this recipe.

2 lbs. fresh green beans

Garlic powder, not salt

2 tbsp. olive oil

Salt and pepper to taste

Clean all green beans and snap in half to get smaller pieces. Heat oil in a pan and when it is hot add the green beans. They should be frying. Cook for 4 minutes and stir twice. Add ½ cup of water and cover. Let them steam about 5-7 minutes. Uncover and stir. Sprinkle 1 tsp. garlic powder over all of the beans, keep frying. Sprinkle ½ tsp salt and ½ tsp pepper on the beans. It is ok if they get a little browned. We don't want them wilted but cooked al dente. Add to the pan you will freeze them in.

Twice Baked Potato Casserole

7 lbs. of potatoes, scrubbed and baked

8 tbs. unsalted butter, plus 1 tbs. separate

1 cup sour cream

2 tsp. salt

½ cup of heavy cream

1 ½ tsp. pepper

¾ lb. bacon cooked crispy and crumbled

½ lb. sharp white cheddar cubed

¾ lb. mild cheddar shredded (3 cups)

½ cup finely chopped chives

3 eggs lightly beaten

Scoop out the baked potatoes and add to a pan. Add butter, sour cream, heavy cream, salt, pepper, and mash together.

Add bacon, cubed and shredded cheese, onions and eggs. Pour into a buttered pan for baking and cover with remaining cheese.

Bake at 350 degrees for 45 minutes. Check to see if cheese is crispy on top. If it is getting dark then cover with buttered foil so it does not stick.

Manwich is just the canned version with fried ground beef. I added this as a change for lunch. I put it into gallon sized freezer bags for easier packing and saving space.

Lasagna Bolognese – I doubled this recipe for the crew

For bolognese sauce:
  1/4 cup olive oil
  3 ounces sliced pancetta, finely chopped
  1 medium onion, finely chopped
  1 large carrot, finely chopped
  1 celery rib, finely chopped
  2 garlic cloves, chopped
  2 pounds ground beef chuck (not lean)
  1 1/2 cups dry white wine
  1 1/2 cups whole milk
  1/4 cup tomato paste
  1 1/2 teaspoon thyme leaves

For Ricotta filling:

> 2 (10-ounce) packages frozen chopped spinach, thawed
> 2 (15-ounce) containers whole-milk ricotta
> 4 large eggs, lightly beaten
> 1/2 cup grated Parmigiano-Reggiano
> 1/2 teaspoon grated nutmeg
> 3/4 cup whole milk, divided

For assembling lasagna:

> 12 Barilla no-boil dried lasagna noodles (from 1 box)
> 1/2 cup grated Parmigiano-Reggiano

Make Sauce:

Heat oil in a 12-to 14-inch heavy skillet over medium heat until it shimmers. Cook pancetta, onion, carrot, celery, and garlic, stirring occasionally, until vegetables are golden and softened, 12 to 15 minutes. Add beef and cook, stirring occasionally and breaking up any lumps, until meat is no longer pink, 6 to 10 minutes. Stir in wine, milk, tomato paste, thyme, 1/4 teaspoon salt, and 3/4 teaspoon pepper. Simmer, uncovered, stirring occasionally, until most of liquid has evaporated but sauce is still moist, about 1 hour.

Make ricotta filling:

Put spinach in a kitchen towel (not terry cloth) and twist to squeeze out as much moisture as possible.

Whisk together ricotta, eggs, parmesan, nutmeg, 1 1/4 teaspoons salt, and 1 teaspoon pepper. Transfer 1 1/2 cups ricotta mixture to another bowl and whisk in 1/4 cup milk; set aside. Whisk spinach into remaining filling with remaining 1/2 cup milk.

Assemble and bake lasagna:
Preheat oven to 375°F with rack in middle.

Soak noodles in a bowl of very warm water until pliable but not softened, 3 to 5 minutes. Place on a kitchen towel (it's not necessary to pat noodles dry).

Spread 1 1/2 cups Bolognese sauce in baking pan and sprinkle with 1 tablespoon parmesan. Cover with 3 noodles, leaving space in between. Spread half of spinach filling on top, then 1 cup Bolognese sauce, and top with 1 tablespoon parmesan and 3 noodles; repeat. Top with remaining Bolognese sauce, 1 tablespoon parmesan, and remaining 3 noodles. Pour reserved ricotta mixture over top and sprinkle with remaining 1/4 cup parmesan.

Cover pan tightly with buttered foil and bake 50 minutes at 375 and test to see how it is cooking. Because the recipe is doubled it may take longer.

Breakfast Casserole (I tripled this for the crew)

8 eggs
4 cups frozen hash brown potatoes
12 oz evaporated milk
2 cups of shredded cheddar cheese
1 tsp. salt
½ tsp black pepper
1 cup diced onion
1 ½ cups diced green and red pepper
1/8 tsp cayenne pepper, more if you like it hotter
1 cup diced ham

Scramble the eggs and evaporated milk in one bowl, add salt, pepper and cayenne to the eggs. Add hash browns, onion, red and green peppers, cheese and ham to the pan it will be cooked in and frozen in. Pour the egg mixture over the hash brown mix. Stir gently, cover in buttered foil and bake at 350 degrees for 45 – 50 minutes. If you have doubled the recipe or more check it to see if it needs to be cooked longer.

Beef and Rice Casserole (I quadrupled this recipe)

1 lb. ground beef

1 cup cooked rice

1 can cream of chicken soup

¼ cup chopped celery

¼ cup chopped green pepper

¼ cup chopped onion

2 cloves garlic

½ tsp. pepper and salt

½ cup cheddar cheese

½ tsp tarragon

1 tsp paprika

1 hatch roasted chili, (habanero works as well)

1 cup of shredded Muenster cheese – for topping not in the casserole

Brown the beef with salt and pepper. Sauté the celery, onions, pepper, garlic in olive oil. Combine all ingredients in bowl and pour into the pan you will freeze it in. Cover with shredded Muenster top with a buttered foil. Bake at 350 for 30 35 minutes.

Spaghetti and Meatballs

Meatballs:

1 lb. ground beef

¾ lb. of pork

3 cloves garlic minced

¾ cup bread crumbs

2 tbsp. dried basil

¼ cup of grated parmesan

2 eggs

Salt and pepper to taste

Add all ingredients together in a bowl and mix by hand. Roll into 2 inches round balls. Heat olive oil in a fry pan and add the meatballs turning to cook through.

I cheated on the sauce. I used Trader Joe's three cheese pasta sauce. I really like it and it compliments these meatballs. I poured the sauce and meatballs into gallon sized bags to freeze so I could save space.

Dinner Burritos – Two kinds, ground beef and spicy Barbacoa beef

Barbacoa meat for burritos

4 lb roast

1/3 cup of apple cider vinegar

3 tbsp. lime juice

4 chipotle peppers – canned in adobe sauce

½ sweet onion

5 cloves garlic

4 tsp. cumin

2 tsp. oregano

1 ½ tsp. salt

1 ½ tsp. black pepper

1/8 tsp. ground clove

1 cup chicken broth

3 bay leaves

Heat oil in a pan, when it is hot add the roast to it and

brown on all sides. Blend all of the other ingredients together. Put the roast into the slow cooker and pour the liquid over them. Cook on high for 1 hour and then drop to low setting. Cook for additional 5 hours turning every hour. After it has cooked and cooled shred it to add to the burritos.

Ground beef was cooked by using a taco seasoning packet and following the directions.

Cilantro Lime Rice to add to burritos (tripled for the trip)

1 tbsp. oil

2 tsp. fresh cilantro

1 fresh lime

½ tsp. salt

1 cup rice

2 cups of water

Sauté rice in a pan with the oil. Add water and cook the rice. When it is cooked mix in salt and lime juice, fluff the rice. Add cilantro after that.

Corn for the burritos

Cook three frozen 12 packages of frozen sweet corn.

Add to the corn 3 chopped jalapeno peppers, juice from 3 limes, salt and pepper.

Set out the two meats, rice, shredded cheese, heated refried beans, large burrito tortillas, sour cream, chives, chopped tomatoes

Make the burritos adding all the ingredients above, using only one type of meat per burrito. Wrap in foil and label mild or hot. Put burritos in large gallon sized bags for storing.

Chicken Tortilla Soup

2 tbsp. oil

1 small onion diced

2 tsp. garlic minced

2 jalapenos diced

1 head of broccoli chopped small

2 stalks of celery chopped

1 red and 1 green pepper chopped

6 cups of chicken broth

1 (14.5 oz) can of fire roasted tomatoes

1 (14.5 oz) can of black beans rinsed

3 cooked chicken breasts

2 limes, juiced

1 tsp cumin

1 tsp chili powder

½ tsp dry oregano

1 cup chopped cilantro

one 8 inch tortilla chopped into strips

shredded cheese

Add oil to a pan and add all the vegetables, stir and cook for about 5 minutes. Add broth, tomatoes, beans and all of the spices. Cook for another 30 minutes covered. When it is cooked uncover and add the chicken, cilantro, lime juice and tortilla strips. The cheese is to be added after it is heated up again. I stored this in gallon sized bags for easier storing.

Acknowledgments:

I would like to thank everyone who helped me work through the project. It truly made the event mean so much more to me. I was very nervous about not having enough food and not having anyone like it but it all worked out well and no one got sick!

To the brave folks who find a passion to race away from land and brave the elements all for the love of sailing!

I would like to thank Bill Helvestine for shining the light before me and passing on amazing advice. Also, the entire crew of Deception, the brave souls who ate the food, Mark Van Selst, Steve Meyers , Jasper Van Vliet, Michelle Sumpton, and Peter Shumar.

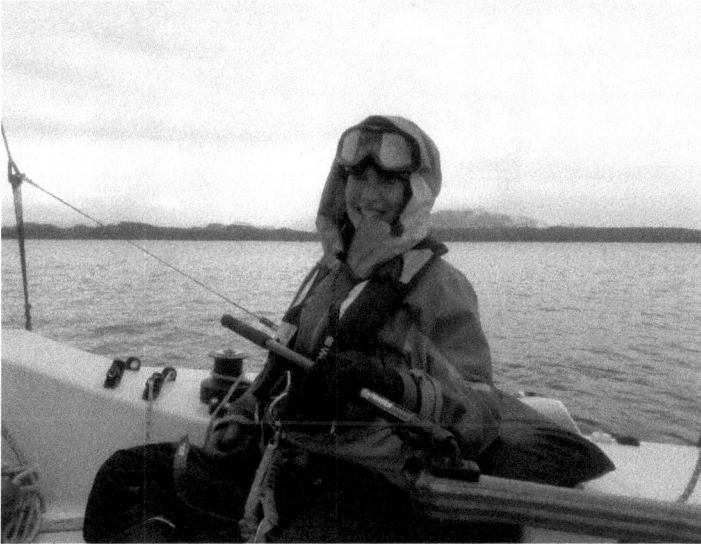

IT'S COLD SOME DAYS R2AK

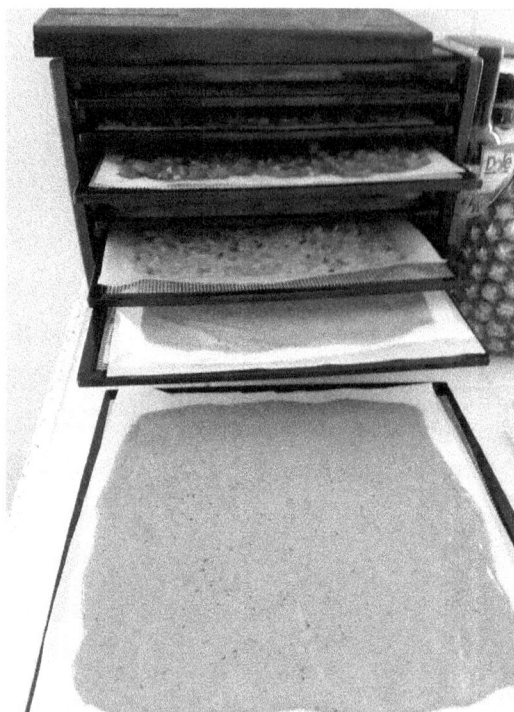

EXAMPLE OF YOGURT DEHYDRATING

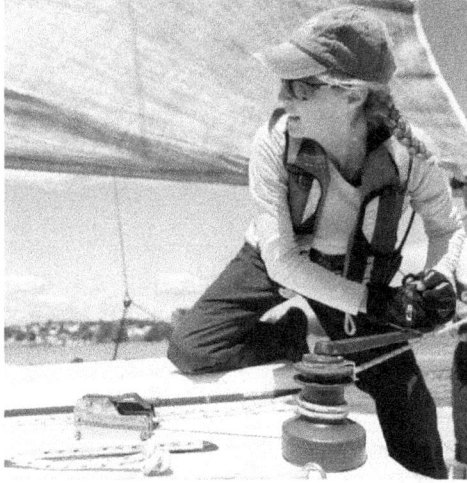

PHOTO BY LIV VON OELREICH, LIVUNTETHERED.COM
AUTHOR UNDERWAY 2ND LEG R2AK

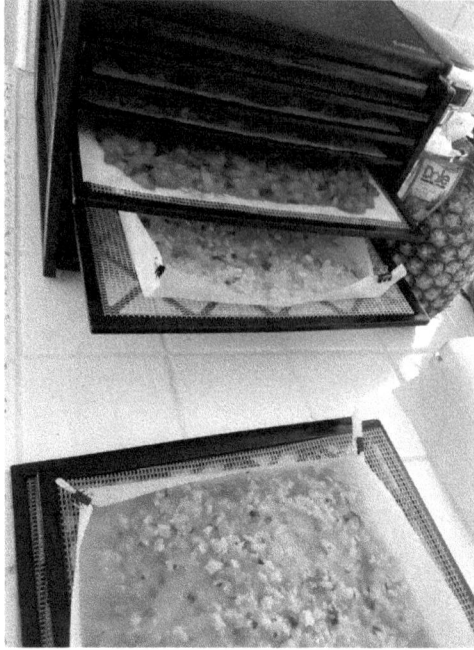

THIS IS HOW YOU DEHYDRATE SOUPS AND STEWS

ABOUT THE AUTHOR

As a profession Stephanie works with corporate executives and business owners as the founder of DES Coaching.com (Don't Ever Stop) since 2008. She believes if you are coaching others on goals and motivation then you should find it for yourself. She grew up on a farm in Ohio around horses and never dreamed she would one day love sailing. After years of chasing opportunities to crew on sailboats in the Channel Islands area of California she was lucky enough to partner with a TransPac crew in 2011 to learn big ocean cooking. Then after pursuing more sailing she got the invite of a lifetime to be on Sistership going for the R2AK in 2017. Life is about going after what you are passionate about!

She currently lives on a sailboat half the year in Mexico with her husband Mark. If you have any questions please feel free to send an email to slyohio@hotmail.com. We all get by with help from others. Good luck!!!

www.ingramcontent.com/pod-product-compliance
Lightning Source LLC
Chambersburg PA
CBHW070819050426
42452CB00011B/2109